Grasping Beautiful

Lessons on life, love and lipstick

by

Stephanie Connors

&

Jessica Guadalupe

Disclaimer: No part of this book is intended as medical advice. The authors are not connected in any way to the medical field. Content is strictly for informational purposes only. Any products mentioned are based solely on the authors' experiences. No compensation has been made from any manufacturer to the authors. Before starting this program, as with any program, it is advisable to consult your physician.

To women
in general and by name,
of all ages and all sizes,

to those happy and healed,
yet yearning for more

to those full of regrets,
wounded, or forgotten

to those who are good,
or pretend to be, or fall in pursuit

to those who are striving, and to
those who have given up

You are known, you are loved,
you are beautiful

Preface
by
Stephanie Connors

Like most women, I have struggled over my lifetime with my external beauty. The highs and lows that began in my teen years are trying to resurface in mid-life. From conversations and observations, I know I am not alone in this journey.

Many childhood and adolescent experiences shaped my thoughts about beauty; some affirming, some painful, all an imprint.

We all have examples tucked away. We believe they are too secret to share; too deep, or too painful. But what if revealing them would bring healing? What if expressing them would set us free?

Let's try. I'll go first.

As hard as I press forward, it is often the painful memories that stick. One comes quickly to mind: the evening my family dined at a local restaurant where the servers gave young patrons thank you toys at the end of the meal. This particular night, I finished off a plate of rigatoni (my go-to choice), and then I sat eagerly awaiting my prize alongside my brother and sister. There she stood at the end of our booth. Our waitress cleared our table, delivered the check and distributed the treats accordingly. To my surprise, and embarrassment, she gave me a truck. Not a pink mirrored compact or a doll or any other girly trinket. I got a truck. I was crushed.

If you were born in the '90s or later, this might not seem like a blow. But in the '70s, when almost *every* store bought item was color coded by gender in either blue for boys or pink for girls, this seemingly innocent error hurt badly.

Confidence shaken, I licked my wounds and vowed to fix my problem. I scoured the pages of every beauty magazine I could lay my hands on. In those days, the pages were filled with celebrities like Farrah Fawcett, Marie Osmond and Brooke Shields. I followed every tip and trick they offered us tweens. And soon I forgot all about that silly old truck toy. Or did I? Did that experience weave its way into how I see myself? Or how I think the world sees me?

Your turn. What is your story? What areas do you struggle? Who in your life can you trust to open up and grieve these times?

Fast forward. Today, I wear joy. I live victoriously. I *grasp* beautiful. You can too. The road was not easy, and I have setbacks now and again. But my *why* for this project is you. If there is any knowledge I have picked up along the way, it is yours in these pages.

Be blessed friend. We are in this together.

Introduction

by

Stephanie Connors

Let's begin. We are so excited - and honored - that you picked up this book. You hold in your hand an opportunity to make a change. A shift in thinking and believing that will not only reshape your life, but those around you.

Our hope is that you come away from this experience healthier in body, mind and soul. And as you walk in this new health, you sow what you learn into others. Please know that we are on this journey with you. Jessica and I have each been transformed in one way or another, and we are eager to share what we have learned along the way.

How about you? Are you ready? Are you willing to start fresh, work hard, dig deep? This coming year is going to fly by like any other year. How do you want this year to differ from the rest? What are your visions and dreams? If you want this year to stand apart, to be significant and purposeful, make the commitment. Choose this moment in time to make the decision. Go for your goals. Do not look back.

We are so glad you are here! We pray the tools in this book will bring you a renewed mindset, personal victories and peace. The book is divided into 12 chapters designed for you to focus on one chapter per month for one year. We tackle the hard topics all women struggle with: worth, value, body image, emotions, aging, makeup, haircare, skincare, fashion and more. Each chapter covers one of such topics. The program works best in order, as the subject matter is primarily cumulative.

Every chapter is then divided into two sections. The first section points to the spiritual aspect of that particular topic. The second section follows up on the spiritual aspect and adds very practical and hands-on exercises to compliment that topic. An area for journaling completes each chapter to help you process your thoughts as you move through the book.

I write the first section of each chapter, while Jessica Guadalupe writes the second *boot camp* section of each chapter. Following this introduction is our **author biographies** so you can learn more about us as women and writers. We hope our backgrounds and ministries will help you apply the material to your life and meet your needs.

Well, it is up to you now. Will you set aside these 12 months to care for your body, mind and soul?

You can begin ANY month of the year. Even if it is mid-year, or late in the year, do not let that deter you. Make your *want to* bigger than any reason to delay. We are here for you! You ARE up for this challenge!

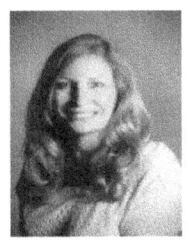 Raised in Pittsburgh, Pennsylvania, **Stephanie Connors** is a Christian author and speaker. A graduate of University of Dayton, Ohio, Stephanie now lives with her husband, Kevin, and two children, Michael and Abigail, in sunny Florida. From personal experience, Stephanie knows God's ability to change a life. Her work includes a wide variety of genre focusing on marriage, parenting and relationships:

- Fiction: **Sew Sisters**; *A Pattern for Hope and Healing*
- Non-Fiction: **The Beautiful Blended Life**; *How to Create a Blended Family that Loves and Lasts*
- *Children's Book: **Know that I Love You**
- Devotional: **Fireside**; *Devotions for the Heart and Hearth*
- Newest Release co-authored with Jessica Guadalupe: **Grasping Beautiful**; *Lessons on Life, Love and Lipstick*

The mission through all Stephanie's writing is for readers to come to know God or grow closer to God through a relationship with Jesus Christ. Many of her books include study guides or journals designed for personal use, small groups, counseling or classes. For speaking arrangements, please contact Stephanie at: stephanieannconnors@gmail.com

You may follow her work on social media at:

Facebook: @connorswrites

Instagram: @stephanieannconnors

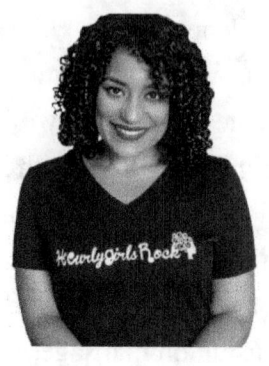

Jessica Guadalupe is a native of Brooklyn, New York. She is a certified minister under the Assemblies of God. She is currently First Lady and Associate Pastor alongside her husband at Rebirth Church in St. Augustine, Florida. From the fruit of their love and blessed union was born their awesome son, Anthony Josiah.

Lady Jess and her husband Rev. Anthony Guadalupe arrived at Rebirth Church in August 2012. Through their ministry, the church has seen incredible growth in every area; including R.I.S.E., Lady Jess's ministry for women.

Gifted at a very young age with a singing voice, she has a passion for worship through song. She is the lead vocalist of the Rebirth Worship Team, and has also led worship at countless events and conferences. Through worship and the unerring Word of God, Lady Jess is earnest in sharing her prayers for revival in St. Augustine and Jacksonville, Florida.

Anyone who has had the privilege to fellowship with Lady Jess would hear how she has, with the grace of God, overcome many obstacles, including insecurity and fear. She testifies how she struggled with these issues for many years, but thanks God for His power and amazing grace.

Her life's theme is found in this scripture: *"Death and life are in the power of the tongue: and they that love it shall eat the fruit thereof."* (Proverbs 18:21 KJV). She has learned that *life* words manifest a life of joy, peace and abundance in the midst of it all. Lady Jess is now a bold and courageous woman of God who yearns for God's presence at all times; a woman who hungers to see women live their purpose and not allow fear and insecurity to dominate them.

Lady Jess is also an aspiring YouTube Vlogger. She promotes natural haircare and helps direct people who would love to embrace their natural hair without heat. She also films makeup tutorials and product reviews. Follow Lady Jess on social media:

YouTube: www.youtube.com/ladyjessg

Instagram: LadyJessG

Facebook: LadyJessG

Twitter: LadyJesg

"Love the Lord your God with all your heart and with all your soul and with all your mind and with all your strength." (Mark 12:30 NIV).

Table of Contents

Heart

There is no better place to start discussing beauty than with the heart. For life itself begins and ends with a single heartbeat. And it is here where the secret to your beauty lies.

Where there is love, there is beauty. Start here. Persevere here. Abide here. You are never more beautiful than when you are in the throes of love. The depth and authenticity of your love reveals your heart. And it is the condition of your heart that determines your beauty.

Let's start with a good hard look at ourselves and examine our hearts. (Remember, I am in this boat with you. I need to examine and reexamine myself *all* the time.) Does the thought of extending a helping hand to a friend cause you stress? Does folding your family's laundry make you bitter? Do you dread sharing a bedtime with your husband?

If you answered yes, (or almost yes), to one or more of these questions, you are not alone. Instead of beating yourself up over these feelings, use them as a signal that you need to refuel. Do not brush them aside; do not stew in guilt. Take action.

In order to be loving, (and thereby beautiful), you must be filled with love. You can only give away something you have. To give love, you must have love, feel loved, BE loved. There needs to be an abundance of love in your heart and spirit to be able to love fervently and consistently. Giving out of overflow is the key to giving genuine, sustaining love.

You must fill up your own love tank. Be deliberate. Be intentional. It is your responsibility; and it should be your highest daily priority. I know, I know that you are thinking: *"I can't. I don't have time." "That is so selfish."* Quite the opposite is true. Filling yourself up with love, so that you have more than enough to give away, is anything but selfish. Remember, overflow happens when you cannot contain what you hold inside. It MUST come out. The only one who can fill you with this kind of love is God. Why? Because *"....God is love."* (1 John 4:8 KJV). If you want to be more loving, spend time with God (love). Let His spirit infuse your spirit. How? First, you must have a relationship with God. And that relationship begins the moment you accept Jesus as your personal Lord and Savior. *"Jesus told him, 'I am the way, the truth, and the life. No one can come to the Father except through me.'"* (John 14:6 NLT).

Before we delve deeper, before we cover any more material, let's lay a foundation for change, or repair a foundation that is worn and weary. A foundation to build upon in this life and secure *eternal* life.

The truth, the TRUTH, is God loves you. No matter where you are at, where you have been, or what you have done, God loves you.

We are all sinners. The Bible says, *"For all have sinned, and come short of the glory of God."* (Romans 3:23 KJV). Sin separates us from God. The Bible says, *"If we confess our sins, he is faithful and just to forgive us our sins, and to cleanse us from all unrighteousness."* (1 John 1:9 KJV).

God provides a way to restore our relationship with Him. God sent His son Jesus to the earth to pay the price for our sins. Jesus willingly died on a cross, was buried, and after three days, rose from the dead and now sits at God's right hand in heaven. *"For God so loved the world, that he gave his only begotten Son, that whosoever believeth in him should not perish, but have everlasting life."* (John 3:16 KJV).

There is a choice for you to make now. The opportunity to build or repair that foundation is set before you. The Bible says, *"That if thou shalt confess with thy mouth the Lord Jesus, and shalt believe in thine heart that God hath raised him from the dead, thou shalt be saved."* (Romans 10:9 KJV).

If you would like to accept God's free gift of salvation, please pray the following prayer to ask Jesus to live in your heart and be your personal Lord and Savior.

Dear God, I am sorry for my sins. I believe that Jesus is your son and that He died on a cross to pay for my sins. I believe that He was buried and after three days he rose from the dead. Please forgive me of my sins and save me. Jesus, I ask you to come into my heart and be my personal Savior and the Lord of my life. Holy Spirit, baptize me, fill me to overflowing with your power and love. Father God, I love you and will live for you all the days of my life. In Jesus' name, Amen

Yes! A resounding yes!! You have made the best and most important decision of your life. **What's next, you ask?**

1) Find a Bible believing, life-giving local church. Plug in. Volunteer, join a small group, take classes.

2) Get a Bible of your own. The church you are attending may have one to gift you as a new believer; or visit a Christian bookstore and purchase one; or find one online. There are many versions these days, so be sure to select a version that speaks easily to you.

3) Set a time and place to read and study your Bible and pray to God. Praying is conversation between you and your Creator. Share your mind and heart. Thank Him, praise Him, ask Him to guide you, and help you in life. Ask Him to fill you with His love.

4) Tell others about your relationship with God and encourage others to meet God and have a relationship with Him through Jesus, too.

5) Live out your faith in everyday ways by loving others in words and deed.

Remember how this chapter started? Well, you have just experienced a makeover, a supernatural makeover. No diet, no surgery, no cosmetics or hair dye can replace God's handiwork. I am so happy for you, *Beautiful!*

Beauty Boot Camp Exercise: Heart

Now that you have chosen to surrender your heart to Jesus, our Lord and Savior, it is very important to protect your heart. In fact, the Bible encourages us to make heart protection our highest priority. *"Guard your heart above all else, for it determines the course of your life."* (Proverbs 4:23 NLT).

There are two ways our heart needs to be protected.....Spiritually and Physically. Let's look now at how we can ensure and maintain that protection.

How do you guard your heart spiritually? The only way we can do anything spiritually is by the guidance and power of the Holy Spirit. The Holy Spirit is a person who dwells inside of us. He is our helper and comforter. We have to speak to Him daily and ask Him to equip us to guard our heart from the snares of the enemy, from confusion, distractions, lies, negative talk, negative people, unhealthy relationships and our own personal will.

The Holy Spirit is our gatekeeper. We have different gates in our lives: the ear gate, mouth gate and mind gate. When we allow the Holy Spirit to be our gatekeeper, He will protect those three gates to prevent anything unhealthy from entering our heart.

Every morning, we get a fresh start. *"Great is his faithfulness; his mercies begin afresh each morning."* (Lamentations 3:23 NLT). When you rise, pray and ask the

Holy Spirit for help. *"Holy Spirit, be my gatekeeper. Do not allow anything to harm my heart today. Show me and direct me in this day, so I can be victorious. Amen."*

How do you guard your heart physically? Everything that we ingest/put into our mouth, everything that we apply to our skin (which is the largest organ in your body) and everything that we do to our body affects our heart. It can be positive or negative. Our physical heart is a muscle, and it is special because of what it does. The heart sends blood around our body. The blood provides our body with the oxygen and nutrients it needs.

Knowing our heart is the motor for our blood to flow in our body helps us understand the great need to guard and protect our heart physically. Here are a few healthy heart ideas for you. *Remember, before starting a new fitness or dietary routine, it is best to seek the counsel of your physician.*

1. **Get Active**. You do not have to join a gym or run in a 5K; however, a 10-15 minute walk a day is a good start. Just begin. Slow and simple. Get your heart pumping so it can flow properly, and then gradually increase the time as you are able.

2. **Eat Better**. Eating the right foods can help you control your weight, blood pressure, blood sugar and cholesterol. Do your best to eat mostly whole foods (food from natural sources), avoid processed foods and limit sugar. Eat what nourishes your body; limit the rest.

3. **Relax**. Take deep breaths, get massages, and find ways to reduce stress. Deep breathing 3-5 minutes a day will help get your blood flowing while regular massages will help relax your mind and body. The idea of massages may bring forth thoughts like, "massages are expensive." However, there are ways to bypass expensive massages. Try having your spouse, child, parent or someone you live with give you a 10-15 minute massage once a week to help you relax. Massage schools have students who need to practice on people. You may be able to get one for free, or for a very reasonable price. A personal masseuse who has a business in their home may charge less than a spa masseuse. Invest in protecting your heart and health in this way; it is well worth it. You are worth it.

4. **Sleep**. Good sleep is essential for a healthy heart. While you sleep, your body replenishes, repairs and restores itself. Proper sleep strengthens your immune system and improves your memory. So, go get some zzzzs. You need it!

We need our heart to survive. Be intentional in guarding it. In His Word, God commands us to guard it. That means it is important to Him. And if it is important to Him, it should be important to us. *"As a face is reflected in water, so the heart reflects the real person."* (Proverbs 27:19 NLT).

Heart *thoughts and jots ~*

_____

_____

_____

_____

_____

_____

_____

_____

_____

_____

_____

_____

_____

_____

_____

_____

_____

_____

_____

_____

_____

_____

Soul

Ask yourself a few questions. How have you been approaching beauty thus far in life? Are you worrying, perhaps obsessing, over a new gray hair or the slightest wrinkle? Are you "white knuckling" through the latest fad diet or exercise trend? Have you had or are you considering some kind of plastic surgery or cosmetic procedure? If you answered "yes" to any of these questions, you are not alone. First, *relax* -- we have all been there! Second, *be open* to a fresh start and a new approach to beauty.

Let's start with a study of ourselves and how we came into being. Understanding *how* you were made will encourage you in life, ease your efforts and allow you to **grasp beautiful**. From the beginning, even before your birth, you were made in the image of God. To gain an assurance of this truth, memorize the following scripture and pray it aloud often -- especially when natural doubts try to creep into your thoughts! *"For you created my inmost being; you knit me together in my mother's womb. I praise you because I am fearfully and wonderfully made; your works are wonderful, I know that full well."* (Psalm 139:13 NIV).

You are essentially a three-part being. You are a **soul** with a **spirit** who lives in a human **body**. The true you, the REAL you, the *innermost* you, is your soul. Your soul consists of your mind, your will and your emotions. Your soul is imperishable and eternal and will live on after your earthly death in either heaven (with God) or hell (apart from God).

Once you place your faith in Jesus, His virgin birth, His substitutionary death on the cross, and His bodily resurrection, your soul is "saved" and will, upon your death, be with God forever. It is at that moment of decision when you accept Christ as your personal Lord and Savior that the Spirit of God (also known as the Holy Spirit) comes to reside in your spirit.

God is a three-part being — just like you!!! He is God, Jesus AND the Holy Spirit, also known as the Holy Trinity. The great mystery is that the Holy Trinity is three separate persons and also one. Looking at your own human makeup will help you understand this mystery. You are spirit, soul and body — all separate parts, but also one.

Your spirit is the part of you that speaks to and hears from God. In essence, your spirit *connects with* God's Spirit. Let's break down the communication process both ways.

How do you hear *from* God? God (through the Holy Spirit) transfers His knowledge to your spirit, and then your spirit transfers that "knowing" to your soul, which expresses itself to the world. Remember, your soul is your mind, will and emotions. So, it is your spirit that *hears* God and it is your soul that *shares* God.

In reverse, how do you speak or pray *to* God? Your soul (mind, will and emotions) speaks aloud or silently the thoughts in your head or on your heart. Those thoughts from your soul are relayed to your spirit, and then your spirit transfers those thoughts to God (through the Holy Spirit). God hears and replies back.

The closer you are to God, the more constant this exchange is in your life. To simplify this exchange, picture a telephone line or internet connection. Think of your spirit and God's Holy Spirit "calling" or "emailing" each other. How exciting! How marvelous! How REAL!!

Now, back to beauty. Your physical body may be the part of you others see with their eyes. But your soul (your mind, will and emotions) is the part of you that others *experience*. Since God is the source of love and all things beautiful, when you express God (express love), you are a beautiful soul and you are authentically beautiful.

So, pick up the original beauty book — the Holy Bible. Spend time with God. Read His Word and "hear" Him speak to you through passages you are reading. How do the words you are reading apply to you and those in your life? Sit quietly, be still and just listen to the silence. It is in that place of peace where God will give you a *specific* direction or answer to prayer. To review, God speaks through the Holy Spirit to your spirit; then your spirit speaks to your soul; then your soul (mind, will and emotions) converts the transmission into corresponding words and actions that the world sees, hears, loves and finds beautiful!

Keep in mind — you cannot force yourself to be loving, and beautiful. Genuine beauty is spirit-led and spirit breathed. Make your goal to be close to God. He *wants* you to feel beautiful, and He will draw others into your life to experience your beauty. For a beautiful soul can lead others to God and a relationship with Jesus and the Holy Spirit. A beautiful soul can encourage a disheartened friend. A beautiful soul can heal a hurting heart. A beautiful soul is for you.

Beauty Boot Camp Exercise: Soul

We learned that our soul consists of our mind, our will and our emotions. The mind, will and emotions are extremely sensitive and powerful at the same time. We have to be intentional of the choices we make with our thoughts and emotions. We, as women, can be very emotional; however, we cannot let our emotions dictate our life. Just because you feel a certain way doesn't necessarily mean it's true. Here are some tips to keep your mind, will and emotions in check:

1. **Morning Prayer.** In the digital world we live in, some of us are tied to our phones (I'm guilty). When we wake up in the morning, we go straight to our phones to check for messages, the weather, news, Facebook, etc. Let's change this routine and try something different and replenishing. As soon as our eyes open, let's talk to God. Let's thank Him for a brand new day, for the privilege to live another day when some weren't able to wake up physically. Let's make some declarations by using the word of God. Let's make ourselves available to the Holy Spirit so He can use us as an instrument on a daily basis. We are called to be His ambassadors. Let's worship Him first thing

in the morning. This will bring such a peace to your spirit, and your spirit will transfer this peace to your soul. Doing this will completely set your mind and emotions on the Lord, and anything the enemy plotted to do to your mind on that day will be cancelled.

2. **Drink lots of water.** Science states that 60-70% of the human body is made of water. Water is extremely beneficial to our bodies. I have read some articles that recommend you drink water first thing in the morning before anything else, because it will give you energy, release toxins and jump-start your metabolism. Drinking lots of water daily will hydrate you, energize you, boost your immune system, promote weight loss, maintain regularity, prevent irritability and mood swings, and help improve skin complexion. Drinking water is practical and very beneficial.

3. **Scalp Massage.** Believe it or not scalp massages are amazing for you. They promote hair growth, help blood circulation, help your nervous system and relax you. Personally, I use an essential oil like lavender or rosemary, adding a few drops to my finger tips and massaging my scalp for 5-10 minutes. It's soothing and relaxing. I recommend a daily 5-minute scalp massage to relax you and promote healthy balanced thoughts and emotions.

Depending on your hair type, you may or may not need to follow up with a shampoo. By using just a few drops of oil, a shampoo is really a matter of preference.

When you surrender your mind, will and emotions to the Lord, you live in peace. It is the will of God that you live in peace. *"Let the peace of Christ rule in your hearts, since as members of one body you were called to peace. And be thankful."* (Colossians 3:15 NIV). He wants us to cast all our cares on Him. Life can be very hard, and if we live by how we feel, we make it harder. Let's focus on yielding to what God wants for us.

Here is a life verse to memorize and keep with you every day. *"And now, dear brothers and sisters, one final thing. Fix your thoughts on what is true, and honorable, and right, and pure, and lovely, and admirable. Think about things that are excellent and worthy of praise."* (Philippians 4:8 NLT.) As we keep our mind on HIM, our thoughts will be flooded with strength and peace.

Soul thoughts and jots ~

Mind

One of the most overlooked, and underrated, aspects of beauty is your mind. As explained in the previous chapter (Soul), your mind is one of the three parts that make up the human soul. To review, your soul consists of your mind, your will and your emotions. Therefore, a beautiful mind is definitely key to a beautiful soul and a beautiful you.

So, how do you beautify your mind? Well, it is not easy. There is no overnight fix. It takes time, consistency, and most importantly, a partnership. You must partner with God, the One who created your mind.

When you first come to Christ, your spirit is regenerated (born again) at once. Your mind, on the other hand, renews little by little, and that renewal requires work on your part. The Holy Spirit, a.k.a the Helper, will be your Teacher. Jesus assures us of this Divine guidance in John 14:26 ESV *"But the Helper, the Holy Spirit, whom the Father will send in my name, he will teach you all things and bring to your remembrance all that I have said to you."*

You must commit time to this transformation. You will have good days, or easy days, and then you will have days full of setbacks. Be patient. And if you start to doubt, remember the Lord's promise in Philippians 1:6 NLT *"And I am certain that God, who began the good work within you, will continue his work until it is finally finished on the day when Christ Jesus returns."*

The best way to create a beautiful mind is to spend time in God's Word. You can do this by reading your Bible or listening to an audio Bible. You should also plug into a local Bible-believing church. Take notes during the sermon, and review your notes midweek while listening to the podcast, if available. The more of God's Word you digest, the more beautiful is your mind. Worry changes to faith, anxiety turns to peace and bitterness becomes love. God instructs in Romans 12:2 NIV *"Do not conform to the pattern of this world, but be transformed by the renewing of your mind."*

What are the topics you struggle with? What negative thoughts plague you? Depression, anger, fear, jealously. Everyone is different. Do not compare yourself to others. Be honest with yourself and dig deep. Get a notebook and write down these topics and their triggers. Find scriptures that speak directly about these thoughts and note them under each topic. (Use a Bible concordance, which is a section in the back of a Bible that lists words or topics followed by scripture references that have that particular word in the verse.) For example: If you have a propensity toward sad thoughts, then search verses with words that would "replace" or "renew" the sad thoughts. Look for perhaps: glad, happy or joy. Keep researching, and reading, and writing. Fill your notebook until the Holy Spirit gives you peace over that thought pattern. Here are a couple joy-filled scriptures you might want to include:

"...weeping may endure for a night, but joy cometh in the morning." (Psalm 30:5 KJV).

"Let all that I am wait quietly before God, for my hope is in him." (Psalm 62:5 NLT).

Next, memorize the scriptures. Post them in your home and car. Let them become an instinctual part of your vocabulary and your very being. And if (when) an old or negative thought tries to creep into your mind, CHOOSE to pull from your reservoir of scriptures. Think them. Say them out loud. Do not dwell on the old negative thought, but instead *"Submit yourselves therefore to God. Resist the devil, and he will flee from you."* (James 4:7 ESV).

Beauty Boot Camp Exercise: Mind

Our mind can be our worst enemy, or it can be our best friend. The Bible speaks about self-control. Proverbs 25:28 (NLT) states, *"A person without self-control is like a city with broken-down walls."* In these times in which we are living, I find that self-control has decreased a great deal. Anxiety, depression, identity issues, discontent, overeating and stress abound. Some feel like they can't control their emotions and their situations, but that's a lie of the enemy.

God gave us self-control, and if He gave it to us, we can use it. Self-control begins in the mind. Speak the Word of God to your mind, and it will change how you feel. You cannot allow your mind to dictate your life. Here are a few steps that have helped me guard my mind.

1. **Speak Life:** In the morning, while you are doing your hair and makeup, turn on some worship music, the Word of God audibly or a sermon on podcast or YouTube and listen to Life words. As you listen, speak them upon your life for *"Death and life are in the power of the tongue…"* (Proverbs 18:21 KJV).

2. **Aromatherapy:** Light a lavender or other aromatherapy scented candle in your room and read an edifying book for your spirit. These aromas are soothing and relax your mind and body. *"Our lives are a Christ-like fragrance rising up to God."* (2 Corinthians 2:15 NLT).

3. **You Time:** It is very easy to neglect ourselves. We are so busy with our home, spouse, kids, job, school, ministry or volunteer work. Someone told me: You can never find time, you have to make it. Go get a manicure, pedicure or a facial for yourself. There's something about taking care of yourself that

increases your endorphins, and you feel good. Groupon has great rates for local spas. There's nothing wrong with investing in self-care (with financial wisdom of course). We work hard and we need to treat our bodies well. The Bible reminds us of this importance in 1 Corinthians 6:19-20 (NIV), *"Do you not know that your bodies are temples of the Holy Spirit, who is in you, whom you have received from God? You are not your own; you were bought at a price. Therefore honor God with your bodies."*

Mind thoughts and jots ~

_____

_____

_____

_____

_____

_____

_____

_____

_____

_____

_____

_____

_____

_____

_____

_____

_____

_____

_____

_____

_____

_____

Strength

If an image of a woman at ideal weight, perfectly toned with six-pack abs comes to your mind, relax. Keep reading. We are going to touch on *physical* strength, as it is important to take care of your body and be at your best to serve the Lord, your family and community. But, the focus of this chapter will be on *emotional* and *spiritual* strength, which God wants to cultivate in us.

With age, comes wisdom (and gray hair, wrinkles and a few extra pounds). And with wisdom comes clarity on what is important and where to concentrate your efforts. As far as physical strength, balance is best. Eat right, exercise often, sleep well and laugh. Maintain healthy relationships, love deeply and keep your word. Be positive, give your best to honorable work, pray and serve. A healthy lifestyle will lay the foundation to be physically, emotionally and spiritually strong.

There may be some who feel this chapter is not for you due to a physical limitation, or perhaps a disability. If you have an illness, or live with chronic pain, the Lord has compassion for you. He loves you dearly. Pray for God to heal you, and He will heal you, *or* give you His strength to live a victorious life in the body He created. Your faith and joy while living with and rising above your condition will be a beautiful testimony. If (or when) discouragement rises up occasionally, turn to God's word for understanding. 1 Thessalonians 5:16-18 (NIV) gives clear and comforting direction: *"Rejoice always, pray continually, give thanks in all circumstances; for this is God's will for you in Christ Jesus."*

At one time or another, everyone will face a physical trial of some kind to a varying degree. The experience, even if it's just the common cold, will zap your physical strength making inner strength even more crucial. Trials are not limited to the physical; there will also be emotional and spiritual trials along the way. Jesus shares this truth (and remedy) in John 16:33 (ESV), *"I have said these things to you, than in me you may have peace. In the world you will have tribulation. But take heart; I have overcome the world."* No matter what trials you have faced in the past, or what lies ahead, peace through Jesus is the means to inner strength.

How? What makes a person strong on the inside? How can you have inner peace in every situation? The answer is the knowledge and application of the Holy Scriptures. Since the Bible teaches that Jesus *is* the Word of God, and since Jesus promises peace *in Him*, then memorizing and drawing scriptures into remembrance must be *how to* have inner peace. To illustrate this teaching, let's examine two verses. John 1:1 (NIV) reads, *"In the beginning was the Word, and the Word was with God, and the Word was God."* John 1:14 (NIV) reads, *"The Word became flesh and made his dwelling among us. We have seen his glory, the glory of the one and only Son, who came from the*

Father, full of grace and truth." Knowing the Bible is inerrant, these two passages tell us that the Word is God and the Word became flesh (Jesus); therefore, the Word is God *AND* the Word is Jesus. And to know the Word is to know Jesus.

Your inner strength comes from a place of peace; and as discussed earlier in this chapter, peace comes from being *in Jesus* (in the Word). Knowing the Word means knowing peace. Knowing peace grows your inner strength. The more Word you know, the more peace. The more peace, the more inner strength. Learn verses that build up your confidence and trust in God, that recharge you and bring you assurance of His love. Once you commit these scriptures to memory, the Holy Spirit will bring them to your remembrance at just the right time.

As with a physical work-out routine, scripture memory must be planned, disciplined and consistent. Your mind, like a muscle in your body, must be exercised regularly to build and maintain its strength. Whether a notebook, flash cards, post it notes or an electronic device, pick your memorization method and apply yourself faithfully and forever. Review, search further, but never stop learning and *"Then you will experience God's peace, which exceeds anything we can understand. His peace will guard your hearts and minds as you live in Christ Jesus."* (Philippians 4:7 NLT).

Beauty Boot Camp Exercise: Strength

I am a big believer in exercise. As the Word of God strengthens our spirits, exercise strengthens our bodies. I believe we all need it, and we all can do it. There are different kinds of exercises and different levels. There is an exercise out there for you.

I had always been overweight since I was a kid. When I was 11 years old, the doctor told my parents that I had high cholesterol and high blood pressure and that was extremely dangerous for me, being so young. They tried putting me on different diets and it was very hard. I was young and really didn't care to lose weight. I felt fine. In my teen years I lost some weight because I began to like boys and wanted to get attention.

When I began dating my husband, we were eating out and late at least three times a week. I was in my 20s and weighed close to 200 pounds. On my wedding day, my dress fit tight because I gained weight instead of losing it. I was an emotional eater, and I made lots of excuses on why I couldn't exercise. I had our son when I was 25, and I didn't like what I saw in the mirror. I also wasn't feeling good. I was short of breath all of the time and feeling lethargic and moody. I knew I needed to make a decision.

I began a weight-loss program with no exercise. I did lose weight; however, after two years of the same thing I plateaued.

My friend who is very knowledgeable on fitness shared with me that I needed to exercise. I gave him excuses up the wall of why I couldn't exercise. He told me that if you want to strengthen your body, you must exercise; and that your mind and body will tell you "no", but that you CAN do it. Start slow and increase gradually.

I joined a gym, and he began to teach me how to breathe while I jogged. When I used to jog, I would get pain in my side and felt nauseous very fast, because I was breathing incorrectly. When I incorporated exercise into my life, my body changed. I was losing weight faster (still on an eating plan), and my body was strengthening. The more I exercised, the stronger I became. I also changed the way I ate and followed healthy food plans while I exercised. Today, twelve years later, I can now jog three miles straight without stopping and went from a size 16 to a size 6. If I can do it, anyone can.

Exercising is not only for losing weight. For anyone who doesn't have a weight problem, your body still needs exercise. Your heart, cells, limbs, muscles, joints, etc., need movement. I am not a personal trainer, but I know when I exercise, I feel accomplished, I feel successful. My endorphins are strong, and I feel like I can conquer the world. The Bibles says in Psalm 91:16 (NLT) *"With long life I will satisfy him and show him my salvation."* Let's do our part in this promise and try our very best to take care of our bodies — for ourselves, for our families and for Him.

Strength *thoughts and jots ~*

_____

_____

_____

_____

_____

_____

_____

_____

_____

_____

_____

_____

_____

_____

_____

_____

_____

_____

_____

_____

_____

_____

Body

Most likely, no other topic causes women more angst and fret than this chapter: Body. Well, ladies, you are not alone. There is a good chance that every woman, at one time or another, has gone or will go through a season when she wishes for a different size, shape or build. But, hopefully, that season passes quickly. If you are there now, or have a hunch you may be there again at some point, take some time to gain a new perspective.

Our bodies change so much over the course of a lifetime. Not just height and weight, but hormonal changes, too. From puberty to childbirth to menopause, our bodies are always cycling and creating in one way or another. We are magnificent, beautiful and complex creations! As we study God's Word, we discover that He made us in *His* very image. *"So God created human beings in his own image. In the image of God he created them; male and female he created them."* (Genesis 1:27 NLT).

Just stop and fathom that truth. God created you. That fact alone makes you a masterpiece. Imagine how it grieves our Heavenly Father that we worry, stress and even cry about our bodies. The Lord loves you so much! If (or when) you are tempted to feel bad about your body, think of your Creator and the joy He had creating you. Shift your thoughts to gratitude for your marvelous birth and personal uniqueness. If (or when) the temptation to feel bad about your body reappears, remind yourself of His design and rejoice in your Divine likeness. Try this: When tempted? Remember, rejoice! Tempted again? Rejoice! Tempted? Rejoice! Repeat until your first and *only* thought about your body is to rejoice.

You are of infinite value to the Lord. Leading a healthy lifestyle is a way of loving God. 1 Corinthians 6:19-20 (NIV) helps us comprehend this correlation *"Do you not know that your bodies are temples of the Holy Spirit, who is in you, whom you have received from God? You are not your own; you were bought with a price. Therefore honor God with your bodies."* You honor God with your body by the choices you make in your life. As discussed in previous chapters: eat right, drink lots of fresh water, sleep well, laugh, exercise often, be productive, pray, love God and others. Honoring your body honors God.

Beyond that, remember this earthly body is a temporal "house" for our spirit; and it is our spirit that lives eternally. One day, we will receive a glorified body as described in 1 Corinthians 15:44 (NLT): *"They are buried as natural bodies, but they will be raised as spiritual bodies. For just as there are natural bodies, there are also spiritual bodies."*

Enjoy life, be thankful for your body, take care of yourself, have a Godly perspective, and if (or when) you hear a woman shame her own body or that of another person, share your testimony. Live, learn, love and pass along your lessons. Journey together, sisters.

Beauty Boot Camp Exercise: Body

Knowing the importance of being strong, inside and out, you are ready to take the next steps. How do you begin? These tips will jump-start your life. Stay committed. Have fun. If you take a step back, begin again right away. Share your story.

1. If you haven't done an annual physical, get that done. Call your doctor and get a checkup.
2. Begin to write down what you would like to strengthen in your body. For example, if you need endurance, strengthen your legs and arms in order to strengthen your heart rate, etc.
3. Eat healthier and cleaner. There are so many clean, delicious foods out there now. Do your research. Read the labels.
4. Begin exercising at least 10 minutes a day. Whether it's a 10-minute walk or 10 crunches. Do something.
5. Present your body to the Lord and ask the Holy Spirit for strength to press on in this health journey.
6. Enjoy the journey. You will look back and be so blessed to see where you came from.

Body *thoughts and jots ~*

Skin

Glowing, radiant, fresh (oh, and young) – ahh! These are the adjectives we long to hear describe our complexion. Like any other organ in your body, your skin needs attention and care. In fact, as mentioned earlier, your skin is the largest organ in the body. It protects our internal organs, regulates our temperature and provides a means to feel sensations like touch, heat, pain and cold.

When we take care of our skin, it takes care of us. We may even consider our skin's condition as an indicator of how we are aging. Our genes, climate and air quality all play a part in how our skin ages. And just like our body type, God made us with a particular skin type. The texture, tone and color were all His idea and doing. For that reason, love your skin and everything about it.

The book of Esther describes at length what went into the skincare and beauty regimen of the women of that period, especially those preparing to meet a King in hopes of marriage. *"Before a young woman's turn came to go in to King Xerxes, she had to complete twelve months of beauty treatments prescribed for the women, six months with oil of myrrh and six months with perfumes and cosmetics."* (Esther 2:12 NIV).

Whether you are single and waiting for your "one," engaged, or a longtime married woman, the Lord encourages us to take time for ourselves to look and feel our best – even as much as a year! Using Esther as an example, be intentional about setting aside time for self-care. *When do you take this time?* Try to schedule some time daily, a longer routine weekly and a full-on beauty day once a month. Finding the right products and a comfortable place to "work" is important. Experiment, study product reviews and watch instructional videos on skincare and makeup application.

Jessica Guadalupe, co-author of this beauty book, has an excellent (and FREE) video channel you can subscribe to for practical tips and helpful information on health and beauty. Educating yourself in this area should be part of your overall wellness program. Stop and take a few minutes right now to check out Lady Jess's channel at: www.youtube.com/ladyjessg. Be sure to subscribe, like and share the link.

This chapter, like the rest, has its foundation in the Word of God. Planting seeds of scripture keeps our priorities well-defined, our minds renewed and our spirits sensitive to God's voice. Ask God for guidance on how He would want you to present yourself. Trust Him to provide the wisdom you need and the provision you need. If (or when), you need encouragement, ask the Holy Spirit to give you peace and bring into remembrance verses that call out your beauty and youthfulness. Post such scriptures on or near your mirror. Smile and speak them aloud. Psalm 103:5 (MSG) can jump-start any morning into a song-filled day of praise: *"He renews your youth – you're always young in his presence."*

Beauty Boot Camp Exercise: Skin

In all reality, no one *wants* to grow old; especially women. We want to look young at all costs. As quoted in the Strength chapter, God says in Psalm 91:16 (KJV) that *"...with long life will I satisfy him...."* It's OK to want to live a long life. No one wants wrinkles. I don't. There are things that can help protect our skin. Our face is the first thing people see when they look at us. It's OK to want our skin to look refreshed and rejuvenated.

Here are a few tips to take care of your skin:

1. **Protect** your face from the sun. Exposure contributes to wrinkles and age spots. As we know, the sun can also be harmful and cause skin cancer. Use sunblock for your face every day. Use sunblock for your body also; however, use a higher SPF for your face. If you are going to be outdoors, wear a sun hat or a visor. If you like to sunbathe, skip the face. Trust me when I say, the sun ages the skin. Reapply sunblock every two hours or as directed on the package. For makeup users, apply sunblock *before* your primer and foundation.

2. **Cleanse** your face twice a day. I used to sell Mary Kay a while back and learned a lot about skincare through the company. Most Mary Kay consultants have amazing skin. They are taught to take great care of it. One thing I remember from those days that will stick with me forever is that if you go to sleep with makeup on, it ages your skin exponentially each night. When you are sleeping, your skin is replenishing and rejuvenating. Makeup trapped in your pores does not let your skin breathe and rejuvenate and promotes aging, dullness, acne and, at times, infection. You must cleanse your skin every morning and every night consistently. This will do wonders in maintaining your skin's radiance.

3. **Moisturize.** After cleansing, there are so many other products you can use for your skin. Serums, toners, face oils, repair creams, masks, exfoliators and eye creams. I use all of it and love it. However, I know many just like the basics. Cleansing and moisturizing are the two most essential steps in skincare maintenance. Moisturizing is imperative. Your skin goes through a lot during the day and overnight while you sleep. After a day of work, our skin is dehydrated. After a good night's rest and the skin replenishing itself, it needs hydration. Moisturizing restores and protects your skin. Even if you have oily skin, you need to moisturize. Using a moisturizer helps prevent aging, hydrates the skin, promotes elasticity and

creates a protective barrier from harmful things in the air. As you use the moisturizer, apply it in an upward motion, which promotes good blood circulation.

4. Drink lots of water.

See Beauty Boot Camp Exercise – Soul #2

Skin *thoughts and jots ~*

Eyes

"I will set no wicked thing before mine eyes:...." (Psalm 101:3 KJV). Think of your eyes like a window. You see out, take in information, and then deposit it into your soul (mind/will/ emotions), where it becomes part of your spirit. It makes sense that what you witness with your eyes will become a part of you. Psalm 101:3 draws a very distinct line on what to look upon and what not. *"NO* wicked thing." It does not say "a little bit of wicked" or occasionally "some wicked."

How should you decide? Seek God on what He considers wicked. Certain topics, like "witchcraft," the Bible is clear on and forbids viewing or participation. Other topics, the Bible is silent on leaving the decision between you and the Holy Spirit. A TV show or sport may be perfectly fine and enjoyable, but be mindful not to let it become an idol in your life. If the TV show or sport comes before the Lord, or interferes with church fellowship, then it is an idol. God commands in Exodus 20:3 (ESV) that *"You shall have no other gods before me."*

With modern technology and divine discipline, you can free yourself of these idols. You can research content to find wholesome choices. You can record TV shows so *you* control your leisure time instead of *it* controlling you. Make this command a natural part of your lifestyle. Your eyes will sparkle and shine, and be beautiful – from the inside out. *"The eye is the lamp of the body. If your eyes are healthy, your whole body will be full of light."* (Matthew 6:22 NIV).

Beauty Boot Camp Exercise: Eyes

Our eyes are very sensitive spiritually and physically. Physically, we use our eyes for everything except sleep. Our eyes need rest. Being intentional in protecting our eyes physically is important.

Here are a few tips I've learned…

1. **Wear sunglasses.** Sunglasses create a protective barrier against the sun. Sunrays can be very harmful to your eyesight.

2. **Eat Healthy.** Eating healthy promotes great protection for your eyes. Carrots have been a popular vegetable for the eyes, but there are many more beneficial foods: Leafy greens and green vegetables (antioxidants), fish (omega-3s), citrus fruits (Vitamin C), eggs (lutein and Vitamin A), carrots and sweet potatoes (Vitamin A/ beta-carotene).

Under-eye protection is also great to help with dark circles, sagginess and puffiness. Using an under-eye cream every morning and every night after you moisturize is very beneficial to your skincare routine. There is a specific way to apply under-eye cream. You need to use your ring finger to dab eye cream under your eyes. The skin under the eye is very delicate and it's the first area of the skin that shows aging. You need to handle it with extra care. The ring finger is the weakest finger on our hands. Using your ring finger helps you apply the cream gently, without being harsh on that area. Gently dab the eye cream under your eye, and you can also give yourself light under eye massages to promote good blood circulation around that area.

I have another eye area tip for those wanting their eyebrows and eye lashes to grow. Using Jamaican Black Castor Oil, aka JBCO, is amazing for hair growth. You can clean an old mascara brush and use it to brush JBCO onto your eyebrows and eyelashes every night. You will begin to see fuller eyebrows and growth on your lashes. It works.

"Look straight ahead, and fix your eyes on what lies before you." (Proverbs 4:25 NLT).

Eyes thoughts and jots ~

Mouth

The Word has so much to say about our mouths – mostly about how we use it. The words that come out, the meaning behind them and even the words we hold back. Never underestimate the weight of your words. They either heal or harm. The Lord clearly explains the consequences in Proverbs 18:21 (KJV), *"Death and life are in the power of the tongue:...."*

Words, at their core, are a heart issue. A person's words indicate the condition of their heart. A beautiful mouth comes from a beautiful heart. God makes it so plain in Luke 6:45 (NLT), *"A good person produces good things from the treasury of a good heart, and an evil person produces evil things from the treasury of an evil heart. What you say flows from what is in your heart."*

Your words are so important and meaningful to our Heavenly Father. They are how you thank, praise and worship Him. The Bible is full of scriptures on the mouth, tongue and lips. Read, meditate and memorize them to understand and prioritize this area of your life — and your beauty.

Jesus makes clear the consequences of our word choices in Matthew 12:36 (ESV) *"I tell you, on the day of judgment people will give account for every careless word they speak."* You will slip. Confess, repent and begin again. The Word contains so much wisdom. *"My dear brothers and sisters, take note of this:*

Everyone should be quick to listen, slow to speak and slow to become angry." (James 1:19 NIV). Learning and living this verse can be a turning point in your life and relationships. You will be obeying God. You will be happier, and definitely more beautiful.

And when you are happier, you shine, you radiate and you SMILE. Yes, your smile is perhaps the most telling feature about you. Your smile is the outward expression of your disposition and attitude. A smile brings joy to others, can change the atmosphere in a room and is simply contagious. Remember, *"A merry heart maketh a cheerful countenance...."* (Proverbs 15:13 KJV).

Beauty Boot Camp Exercise: Mouth

"Righteous lips are the delight of a king, and he loves him who speaks what is right." (Proverbs 16:13 ESV0.

Our mouth is an instrument. We can use this instrument for great things; however, we must take care of it. Exercise excellent dental health by brushing and flossing several times a day, and as well as routine checkups. Getting your teeth and gums cleaned by a dentist every six months is imperative. Dental issues can be extreme in all aspects: extremely dangerous, painful and expensive. Always be attentive to your breath. It is ideal to carry breath mints, gum, breath strips, or even a mini toothbrush and toothpaste. We should always want our breath smelling fresh.

I love to exfoliate my lips. It's an extra step to my skincare routine; however, it is so beneficial. If you use lipsticks, lip-glosses or liquid lipsticks, you definitely need to exfoliate. Our lips need hydration and deep cleaning. Exfoliating your lips removes dead skin and replenishes your lips. A quick DIY recipe for a lip exfoliator is mixing 1 tablespoon of raw honey and 1 teaspoon of granulated sugar (not powdered) together to create a lip scrub. I recommend exfoliating twice a week. After you exfoliate your lips, use a lip balm to moisturize. You will feel the difference instantly. Your lips will be soft, clean and hydrated.

Lipstick is always a good idea. I find that when I wear lipstick, my confidence rises. This doesn't mean that lipstick represents me, but it's just an enhancement to me. I love a nice matte neutral brown lipstick, but I also love bold and fun colors. There are so many different types of lip products in the beauty market. Go pick up something that is fun and bold and pucker up.

Mouth/ Teeth/ Lips thoughts and jots ~

Hair

"....but if a woman has long hair, it is her glory? For her hair is given to her for a covering." (1 Corinthians 11:15 ESV). Now, this scripture may conjure up all sorts of mental pictures, as well as feelings of confusion, guilt or even pride. Let's explore what the Bible says about hair and hopefully set your mind at ease.

Like every other part of the body, your hair is unique to you. God has created hair in a rainbow of colors and textures. He has given some curly hair, some straight and some in between. Some folks' hair grows fast, while others hair seems not to grow at all. For starters, accept your uniqueness, and be content. It seems like people want what they do not have themselves. If you are born with curly hair, you crave straight and vice versa. To covet another's locks is not only sin, but it will detract you from knowing your worth and throw you right into the dangerous and unhealthy comparison trap.

In the Bible, Paul devotes much teaching to gender roles and differences. Some are specific to the time and culture, but there is much to glean and apply to today. The point and overall theme of Paul's teaching would be that women (and growing girls) should be feminine and different in appearance to men. And one of the most obvious ways to show this difference is in hairstyle.

Clean, well-maintained, age and lifestyle is a good starting place for choosing a hairstyle. Changing your style, length or even color can be just plain fun and bring a lift to your spirit. And when your spirit is light, your disposition is cheery, and you are naturally beautiful.

Now a word to the wise, aka, mature readers. I, for one, am so happy that the Lord included Proverbs 16:31 (NLT) *"Gray hair is a crown of glory; it is gained by living a godly life."* It is inevitable. You will get gray hair, and your hair will thin. Enjoy your luscious locks while you are young. Experiment and have fun with different cuts and styles. No regrets. Then, as you mature, embrace the change and live it.

The time will come in almost every woman's life when she will consider not coloring, and explore the idea of letting her hair go completely gray, or white. I am not an expert in that process (yet). And I keep pushing up the deadline each decade. Who knows? I may just keep right on coloring, but then again, I might stop tomorrow. I guess what I am trying to say is that it is a very, VERY, personal choice. Consult the Lord, pray, and then go full on — either way. My hunch is that the Lord would desire us to age gracefully, including our hair, or he could have just omitted that sweet verse in Proverbs.

If you have a medical condition that has caused you to lose some or all of your hair, take heart. You are not alone. Hormone imbalances, thyroid conditions, menopause, and, of course, cancer treatments are among the causes of hair loss. There are doctors, stylists and charitable organizations that can help. Be brave. Find a friend. Explore your options.

Lastly, remember, when you are comfortable being authentic and true, you will *feel* beautiful and *love* beautifully.

Beauty Boot Camp Exercise – Hair:

For those who know me, they know hair has become my passion. November 10, 2017 was my four-year anniversary of going natural. What does that mean? Well, it means that I have naturally curly hair and for many years, I straightened my hair because I desired pin-straight hair. All of the years of using heat to straighten my hair damaged my curly locks and made my texture very fine. Four years ago, I saw a video of a girl who restored her curls. She shared her journey on how she did it, and I was totally convinced. I was tired of my damaged hair. I completely gave up heat on my hair. I also made the choice to not color it. I began changing my hair products and investing in clean ingredient products. I watched lots of videos on how to maintain your natural hair. I take care of my hair like it was a baby: gently and lovingly. I've embraced my curls, and I can say "I Got My Curls Back." It was a long journey, and it's still a journey, because I dedicated myself to care for my hair this way forever.

Many women are not satisfied with their natural hair and it's my goal to help them embrace what God has given them. All of our hair is unique in its own way. My curl patterns are not the same. I have different curl patterns and some curls need more care than others. It's amazing how God created us. *"... even the very hairs of your head are all numbered."* (Luke 12:7 KJV). His creativity and art in creating us is so amazing. Embrace your hair; take good care of it.

One of my favorite tips that I want to share is scalp massages. Every night before I go to bed, I give myself a scalp massage with an essential oil blend I make. You can use coconut oil, jojoba oil or olive oil (just a few drops), and if you want your hair to grow add a drop or two of Jamaican Black Castor Oil (JBCO) to the oil of your choice. I add a few drops to my fingertips and begin massaging my scalp for 5-10 minutes. It's very relaxing, soothing and promotes hair growth. I look forward to my scalp massages every night. I've seen great results with this practice, and I believe it's for any type of hair. If your hair is very oily, jojoba oil is very light and shouldn't weigh your hair down; though some may need to follow up with a shampoo in the morning.

__Hair__ thoughts and jots ~

Nails

I have experienced all the extremes of nail "fashion." From acrylic nails and tips to gel nails (my favorite) and even press-on nails – I have tried them all. Currently, I am enjoying rounded, medium length fingernails, with only a clear, strengthening top coat and pretty baby pink on my toenails! I actually LOVE to have my nails done — my toenails especially. How about you? I guess I do not see it as a necessity, like dental hygiene or basic haircare, but there is just something about have manicured hands and feet. Painted nails are a simple luxury to me. I like to look down at my hands and feet and see the pretty colors.

Also, beautiful nails are memory-making to me. I have had many relaxing times in a salon, sometimes alone, sometimes with a friend, but always, ALWAYS a pleasure. And at home, I have such sweet memories sitting with my sweet daughter and "doing nails" together. Just the two of us, chatting, complimenting each other's color choice or fun designs.

I think what I really like about having nice nails is that I do not have to look in the mirror to see this "artwork." There is no combating any negative self-talk, or "wishing" for this or "wishing" for that. Just glance down and enjoy.

Our nails, ultimately our hands and feet, are most beautiful when they are used to serve the Lord, family, our church and our community. God is good! He encourages us so much in His

Word. *"And how are they to preach unless they are sent? As it is written, 'How beautiful are the feet of those who preach the good news!'"* (Romans 10:15 ESV). Bringing the gospel to others requires travel, whether it is across the street or across the globe. Use your feet for His glory. The Lord makes it clear here. Beautiful feet, go.

God also speaks specifically about our hands and arms in Scripture. Proverbs 31 gives examples of helping hands, outstretched arms, hardworking hands and loving arms. *"[10]A wife of noble character who can find? She is worth far more than rubies. [11]Her husband has full confidence in her and lacks nothing of value. [12]She brings him good, not harm, all the days of her life. [13]She selects wool and flax and works with eager hands. [14]She is like the merchant ships, bringing her food from afar. [15]She gets up while it is still night; she provides food for her family and portions for her female servants. [16]She considers a field and buys it; out of her earnings she plants a vineyard. [17]She sets about her work vigorously; her arms are strong for her tasks. [18]She sees that her trading is profitable, and her lamp does not go out at night. [19]In her hand she holds the distaff and grasps the spindle with her fingers. [20]She opens her arms to the poor and extends her hands to the needy. [21]When it snows, she has no fear for her household; for all of them are clothed in scarlet. [22]She makes coverings for her bed; she is clothed in fine linen and purple. [23]Her husband is respected at the city gate, where he takes his seat among the elders of the land. [24]She makes linen garments and sells them, and supplies the merchants with sashes. ²⁵She is clothed with strength and dignity; she can laugh at the days to come. ²⁶She speaks with wisdom, and faithful instruction is on her tongue. ²⁷She watches over the affairs of her household and does not eat the bread of idleness. ²⁸Her children arise and call her blessed; her husband also, and he praises her: ²⁹Many women do noble things, but you surpass them all. ³⁰Charm is deceptive, and beauty is fleeting; but a woman who fears the LORD is to be praised. ³¹Honor her for all that her hands have done, and let her works bring her praise at the city gate. "* (Proverbs 31:10-31 NIV).

When you consider this poem, you may be inspired; you may be challenged or maybe even overwhelmed. Each woman probably interprets the chapter differently, depending on her season of life and how well she feels she is living her calling. Know this: God loves you. He wants the best *for* you, and He wants the best *from* you. The overarching theme of Proverbs 31 is **not** to try in your own might to accomplish ALL the tasks like a "to do" list, but rather to be vigilant and tenacious to be the best YOU in whatever role God places you into in life. So, hands down – God loves you, *Beautiful!*

Beauty Boot Camp Exercise: Nails

I have a confession to make: I bite my nails and have since I was a little girl. I blame it on my big sister. She used to bite her nails all the time, and I was led to do it because of her, right? Honestly, I know it's a bad habit and it's not classy at all. Sometimes, I don't even know that my fingers are in my mouth. My friends tell me "Stop biting your nails," and I am shocked, because I didn't know they were there. That's bad...I know. I still struggle with this habit; however, I found something that has helped. It can be costly but it has helped me. Gel Manicures. I used acrylic tips on my nails for many years but that damaged my nails to the extremes. Gel manicures can weaken the nail beds as well but I find it's not as extreme as acrylics. I love that the nail polish does not come off and I can't bite it off. This has helped my nails grow and look representable. I'm also applying self-control on the nail biting. When I remove the gel manicure and do not get them re-done, I do my own manicure at home. It's not the same quality as the nail salon but I notice when I have nail polish on my nails, I don't bite my nails as much. Your hands are part of your beauty; it's a great idea to keep them clean and pretty.

A pedicure is my best friend. I love it so much. We walk on our feet most of our lives, and they can take a beating. In addition, shoes can hurt our feet. Taking care of our feet should be important also. I've learned to exfoliate my feet while I'm in the shower. We gather a lot of dead skin on our feet that needs to be removed. Scrubbing with a stone and a soap scrub is so beneficial. You will feel instant results. Foot massages are also amazing. They relax you and soothe you and help the circulation of your feet and legs. Sometimes, my son gives me a foot massage, and I use it for quality time with him. He's so sweet.

Our Father desires for us to take care of our temple. All of these tips are suggestions; some may apply or all may apply to use. Use what can benefit you to embrace your beauty from the inside out. Much Love.

Nails *thoughts and jots ~*

Makeup

I have loved makeup for as long as I can remember. Even as far back as elementary school, I loved to dabble in the "arts." Perhaps it was because I danced as a child and got a taste of makeup from having to wear it at the annual recital. For whatever reason, my interest in makeup and products has never stopped. I even tried my hand at a few "stay at home" opportunities selling makeup and skincare. But my "hobby" ate into my profits and I could never make any real money at my business.

Today, I affectionately tell my family that I am going to do my "arts and crafts" (translated that means put on my makeup). One of the pleasures for me personally is that it gives me private time. And during that time, I slowly, ever so slowly, apply my treasures. As much as I enjoy (and perhaps rely) on the color in my clear cosmetic bag, it is the "me" time that really brings out beauty. It is just precious to sit and relax, uninterrupted, for 10 or 15 minutes a day. Whatever the reason, rarely a day goes by that I do not apply my favorites. This is NOT to say this is for you, or the next person, but it makes me happy.

So, to me, it just boils down to this – attitude. Wear what makes you happy. *"Rejoice in the Lord always: and again I say Rejoice."* (Philippians 4:4 KJV). Wear makeup that makes you feel confident and glad. Do not wear it to impress others, or to draw attention to yourself. Use moderation. Stay close to natural, because you were made in the image of God and that image is beautiful – with or without makeup.

When you look in the mirror and begin your application, study your features. Give thanks for your features. Resist the urge to compare, complain or wish for "this or that". Learn to like how you look – with makeup AND without. Particularly if you have daughters, it is important to verbally affirm yourself out loud– especially in their presence. They are watching and will one day be your age and face all the things that you are processing now. If you do not feel like being positive about your appearance, do it anyway. For them!! Commit to this attitude, and soon your positive thoughts will manifest positive words and actions, which will spread to those around you and be passed down through the generations. Be humble, not vain or conceited. Most of all, have a thankful heart for your life, your uniqueness and your Creator.

Another very important aspect of this chapter is staying within your family budget. If you are married, perhaps talk with your husband about a "beauty budget" or allotment for the month that your family can sustain and plug in as a fairly regular number. After the amount is agreed upon, stay in budget. If you are single, pray about it. Have a budget and stick to it as well (which is good practice for marriage one day!) Sure, it is fun to go to the mall and buy the name brands after a "make-over" or consultation, but if it is not practical for your family; there are

MANY drugstore brand equivalents. Jessica will share more on that in her Beauty Boot Camp Exercise.

In the meantime, have fun, experiment and enjoy. Remember to go makeup free some days too (or all the time if you like!). It is really a matter of personal preference. Wear what makes you feel bright, cheery and yourself.

Be good to you! When you are full of love and joy, that fullness will flow outward – to God and to others.

"He answered, 'Love the Lord your God with all your heart and with all your soul and with all your strength and with all your mind'; and 'Love your neighbor as yourself.'" (Luke 10:27 NIV).

Beauty Boot Camp Exercise – Makeup:

"Beauty begins the moment you decide to be yourself..." Coco Chanel. Using makeup is a preference. It doesn't represent who you are as a person. In my opinion, it's a tool to enhance our natural beauty. Some people just don't like makeup or do not know how to use it; therefore, they stay away from it. Some may be allergic to it or may dislike the feeling on their skin. As for me personally, I absolutely love it. Makeup is an art.

As a child, I grew up attending a church that didn't allow women to wear makeup. Unfortunately, we were taught that wearing makeup was a sin. I didn't begin to wear makeup until I was an adult. I had a hidden love for it but respected the rules in my home. When I felt free to wear makeup, I had no idea what to do with it. I just knew the very basics: light eye shadow, black eyeliner on my lower lid, face powder, lip liner and lipstick. That was my basic look for years. Makeup can be intimidating, and I've come to learn that is the reason why many women say they don't like makeup. They are intimidated by how to use it and believe they would look like a clown.

I am a self-taught makeup artist. I learned how to apply makeup through watching YouTube videos, advice from other makeup artists, friends and trial and error. There are so many different makeup techniques and so many different makeup products. I advise you to use products according to your needs. Here are the products I use for my everyday look (it may seem like a lot, but when you get use to using makeup, it's not):

Eyebrow Pencil: To fill in my brows in areas that are sparse

Concealer: To prime my eyelids so my eye shadows do not crease and for my under-eye dark circles.

Eye shadow Palette: I use a base color, crease color and lid color.

Mascara: Love to accentuate my lashes.

Face Primer: To create a protective barrier between your skin and foundation.

Foundation: To even out the skin and cover scars and blemishes.

Face Powder: To set the foundation in place (I just use it on my T-Zone area).

Contour/Bronzer: To bring back some definition to your face.

Blush: Gives you a hint of color on the apples of your cheeks.

Highlighter: To highlight the highpoints of your cheekbones.

Lip Product: I love liquid lipsticks because they are long-lasting.

Setting Spray: This helps set your makeup in place.

Again, everything is to your liking. This is just an example of my everyday makeup routine. I switch it up a lot. You can watch my in-depth tutorials on my YouTube channel www.youtube.com/ladyjessg.

I'm a huge promoter of "Beauty on a Budget." Makeup can be very expensive. High-end makeup prices have become outrageous. I personally use both high-end and drugstore makeup. I have so many drugstore products that I love and have the quality of high-end products. I do not believe you need to buy high-end makeup to have the best makeup look. The beauty industry is booming, and the drugstore brands have picked up their quality. My only preference on high-end products is my skincare products. To save money on makeup, you can watch product review videos. They help a lot. I also add my email to the website of the brand I love, and they send me coupons. I always wait for big sales to stock up on makeup. I rarely ever pay full price on a product. I also clip coupons for drugstore makeup I love. You can double, or triple-up, on coupons and get a lot of makeup deals.

Once again, makeup doesn't represent who you are as a person. Don't feel the need to hide behind makeup. We are gorgeous with or without it. We must embrace our flaws. No one is perfect. Even the airbrushed girls on magazines and on television are not perfect. Technology can do amazing things. My nose is a little big to my liking, and I've learned that I can reduce it by doing a makeup technique called nose contour. I do it for special occasions, but that doesn't mean I hate my nose and can't leave home without hiding it. It's how God made me, and I'm unique in my own way. So are you, *Beautiful*.

Makeup thoughts and jots ~

Clothing, Jewelry and Accessories

Oh, dear! If you were to ask my sweet young daughter, she would tell you that I should just skip this chapter. Yes, it is true. When I need fashion advice, I head straight to her. She has ALWAYS been good at choosing outfits, mixing colors and adding just the right accessory. I, on the other hand, would rather wear what my family affectionately calls "Mom's black dress."

I was always extremely tall for my age growing up; and I was very underweight (although the underweight days are long gone). It was so very difficult to find anything that would fit me, let alone be stylish. I didn't even have a curve to my body until after motherhood. So, the solution: my mom had me shop in the boys' department! Because, you guessed it, the boys' clothes fit. Then, when I really hit a growth spurt, my mom had to get really creative. (I know – the Lord uses these experiences to humble and grow us, right?!) Are you ready? My mom would sew curtain fringe to the bottom of my pants, mostly jeans. Needless to say, childhood was tough at times. But, I survived, thrived and thank my mom for giving me her all. And fortunately, designers have come up with better options these days. Yeah for skinny jeans!

Now that you know some of my fashion background, I am sure you are chuckling and agreeing with my daughter. Well, I have come a long way. I shop in the women's department, of course, and do my best to select comfortable and flattering clothes. At least, I try.

Spiritually speaking, I believe the Lord provides for our needs. Not just food and drink, but clothes also. *"And why do you worry about your clothing? Look at the lilies of the field and how they grow. They don't work or make their clothing, yet Solomon in all his glory was not dressed as beautifully as they are."* (Matthew 6:28-29 NLT).

If you are in a season of financial abundance, then it would be prudent to buy wardrobe staples that are of very high quality that will last should a valley come your way. This season might also be a good time to give back by donating gently used or new (bought and never worn) clothing to an organization whose mission you support.

If you are in a season requiring heavy budgeting, leaving little or no money for new clothing, do not fret — there are options. There are many, many thrift stores that carry very nice clothing. It might not be brand new, but it will be new to you! Also, try a clothes swap with family and friends. Pull out and display all the clothing and accessories that you are no longer wearing. Invite people to come over and do the same. Then shop from each other!! Suggest a limit, perhaps two items per "customer"/ guest. Such a fun way to share and get some new goodies!

Although I might not know a lot about fashion, I do believe the Lord wants us to be modest. We can be stylish and attractive without going too low or too high. Just look in the mirror and be honest with yourself, and if the Holy Spirit prompts you to change, then change.

Now, if you are married, you might consider wearing that outfit for a home date, for an audience of one. *xoxo*. But if you are single, do not give in to any temptation to wear such outfits to lure a date. Although it might bring you attention, it more than likely will not be God's choice for you. Be patient, pray and trust in the Lord's timing for provision. (Yes, in love too). *"Therefore, as God's chosen people, holy and dearly loved, clothe yourselves with compassion, kindness, humility, gentleness and patience."* (Colossians 3:12 NIV).

Above all, ask the Lord for help in *all* things, even shopping and selecting your style of clothing and jewelry. Be fresh and feminine, and remember the best accessory is a smile.

Beauty Boot Camp Exercise – Clothing, Jewelry and Accessories:

If you ask my husband what Jessica's hobby is, he would say SHOPPING!!! I love shopping. You can blame my mommy. My mom blessed me with this hobby. I remember as a little girl, she would take me shopping with her all the time. Our mommy/daughter days were usually shopping. She loved to dress me up and would buy me the cutest dresses and would always tell me how pretty I was and how special I was because she knew that I struggled with not liking my weight. Mommy filled me with *life* words. She was building my spirit, and I didn't even know it until I grew up and recognized how God used her. If she didn't have enough money for both of us, she would only buy for me. Even now when I go visit her in New York, we spend our days shopping. Disclaimer: Window shopping is also considered shopping to me. I don't always come out with stuff, but I just enjoy going to the stores. I'm a frugal spender.

Clothes, jewelry and shoes are my favorite. I love shopping for new clothes and playing around with fashion trends and thinking out of the box. The same way I do not pay full price for my beauty products, I usually do not spend full price for my clothing. I'm a clearance and sale rack girl, and I'm proud of it. I have found that full-price clothes usually go on sale within two weeks. So save your money and wait for sales or look for coupons. An app called RetailMeNot allows you to search for stores and find coupons. You show the cashier the phone, and they scan the app coupon, and you have saved money.

I can be very picky with jewelry. I have more costume jewelry than real gold jewelry. The reasons are: 1. Real gold has become extremely expensive and 2. I lose my jewelry. I change my jewelry every day. I match my jewelry with every outfit. I also love jewelry with beautiful messages on it. I have a beautiful necklace that has the Proverbs 31 verse on it.

Jewelry and accessories can enhance your outfit. A necklace can be a gorgeous statement piece for your outfit. It can make a black dress easily stand out. A scarf can make an outfit sophisticated and classy. A sparkly headband can bring your ensemble to life. It's amazing what accessories can do to your entire outfit. Try something out of your comfort zone on accessories. You may like it.

During the week, I usually dress business casual because I have a corporate job. However, on the weekends I like to dress down but look cute. I love my jeans with holes (nothing too crazy), cute tops and tees, and some cute sneakers or boots. My favorite accessory to wear with my jeans is big hoops earrings. Yes, that '90s look is all me. All I need is to outline my lips with brown lipliner and wear brown lipstick and I'm back to the '90s trend. What's amazing about fashion is that it repeats itself.

Putting together clothing, jewelry and accessories is also an art. You can be so creative with what you have. When shopping is not in the budget, I use what I have but interchange it. I can't tell you how many times people think the outfit I'm wearing is new and it wasn't. I just changed it up with other things in my closet. You can be creative with what you have and rock it.

We should always stay humble in our heart without letting competition, jealously and envy in, because the secular fashion world can create that mindset. However, as believers we do not have to look boring, dull, as if we are suffering. That is a poverty mindset, and we are the children of the King of Kings. We are royalty. *"Trust in the Lord with all thine heart; and lean not onto thine own understanding. In all thy ways acknowledge him, and he shall direct thy path."* (Proverbs 3:5-6 KJV).

Clothing, Jewelry and Accessories *thoughts and jots ~*

Epilogue

We are so proud of you! You are looking and feeling better than ever – and it shows! We pray this time has been a blessing and that you are enjoying life to the fullest!

Now, go. Grab a friend, or two, and gather to discuss what you learned and how you have grown this year. Keep it simple. All you really need is each other.

Be sure to check Facebook for the online **Grasping Beautiful Community** to connect with women just like you (and us).

From our hearts to yours, may the Lord shower you with love, joy, peace, and everlasting beauty.

Stephanie and Jessica